DISCLAIMER/TERMS OF USE

ISBN: 978-1-300-91554-6

Cover Design by Bensmiles

Written by Jimmy Spears

Do you wish to develop healthy habits but find it challenging to do so? Then, you should use this worksheet. Get the hang of forming positive routines and breaking negative ones. Changing your habits and accomplishing your goals in life is possible by applying the methods outlined in the book Atomic Habits.

The purpose of this workbook is to serve as a companion to the source material. This workbook contains action steps that will assist you in putting James Clear's advice into action. This guide is meant to serve as a starting point for creating your system for establishing and maintaining positive routines.

You can improve your life in many ways by putting in the time and effort required to complete the exercises in the workbook.

The worksheet's chapters give you:

• A comprehensive overview

• Insights that are crucial to each chapter

• Insight-provoking queries

• Prospective aims

• Courses of action

    •   The use of to-do lists

I recommend taking stock of your current situation before diving into the workbook. Consider some of your routines right now. Identify both the positive habits you wish to adopt and the negative ones you want to ditch by jotting them down. (The checklist of steps to take is located at the end of Chapter 1.)

Check back with this list as you progress through the workbook and after you've finished it to evaluate which of the tactics and ideas offered here most apply to your situation.

Developing more desirable routines can aid in eliminating undesirable ones.

EXPANDING ON JAMES

Regarding the science of routine, only some people can compare it to James Clear. The New York Times, The Wall Street Journal, and Time magazine frequently feature his work, and he often gives talks at Fortune 500 businesses. Over a million people subscribe to his "3-2-1" email weekly, and millions visit his website monthly.

To aid people and businesses in developing more positive routines, Clear introduced the Habit Academy in 2017.

His best-selling book, Atomic Habits, systematically explains the psychological underpinnings of habit formation. His advice is helpful for both forming and breaking habits of all kinds.

From various vantage points, he demonstrates how to form and break habits.

Atomic Habits is a guidebook for making lasting behavioral changes based on the author's extensive research and study. Good planning, time management, self-discipline, and consistency will allow us to reach our goals if we establish a method for improving by 1% daily.

Personal anecdotes and other real-world examples populate James Clear's book as well.

How often have you considered replacing a negative routine with a more positive one? Was it a challenge for you? Despite our best intentions, it is often easier to maintain a new way once we've established one.

Keeping your new habits and reaching your goals is made easier with the help of the steps outlined in Atomic Habits. By making manageable adjustments to your routine and sticking with them over time, the book and accompanying workbook will show you how to achieve your goals.

The book's central idea is that minor adjustments can significantly impact. Developing positive routines is essential to making lasting changes in one's life. This is a point-driven home throughout Atomic Habits and helpful suggestions for breaking bad habits and forming new, positive ones.

Contents

Disclaimer/Terms of Use... 3

About The Workbook.. 4

    Expanding on James.. 5

Introduction 13

PART ONE:... 15

THE FUNDAMENTALS: WHY TINY CHANGES MAKE A BIG DIFFERENCE 15

Ch 1: The Surprising Power of Atomic Habits 15

    Summary... 15

    Marginal Gains 15

    The Power of 1% Change 16

    The Limitless Potential Plateau 16

    Results, Objectives, and Methodologies... 17

    1. Winners and losers both share the same goal.............................. 18

    2.   A brief change occurs when goals are achieved. 18

    3.   Goals prevent you from being happy 18

    4.   Goals do not promote long-term advancement. 18

    Important Takeaways from This Chapter 19

    Determine Related Problems... 19

    Objectives You Want to Reach... 19

    Your Action Plan... 20

    Action Checklist.. 20

    Example of good habits:.. 21

    Example of bad habits:.. 21

Ch. 2: How Your Habits Shape Your Identity (and Vice Versa)...................... 22

    Summary... 22

    Identity vs. Result... 22

    Change who you are to benefit you... 23

    Important Takeaways from This Chapter 23

Determine Related Problems.. 24

Objectives You Want to Reach... 24

Your Action Plan... 24

An action plan 25

Ch. 3: Four Simple Steps to Creating Better Habits 26

Summary 26

Why do we develop routines? 26

How can we create habits?... 26

The Four Laws of Changing Behavior 28

Important Takeaways from This Chapter 28

Determine Related Problems.. 28

Objectives You Want to Reach... 29

Your Action Plan... 29

Action Checklist.. 29

PART TWO:.. 31

THE 1ST LAW: MAKE IT OBVIOUS 31

Ch 4: The Man Who Didn't Look Right... 31

Summary 31

James offers two methods we might do to become more conscious of our habits: 31

Important Takeaways from This Chapter 32

Identify Related Issues 32

Objectives You Want to Reach... 32

Your Action Plan... 32

An action plan 32

Ch 5: The Best Way to Start a New Habit 34

Summary 34

Application Objective.. 34

Habit-stacking 35

Important Takeaways from This Chapter 36

Determine Related Problems.. 36

Objectives You Want to Reach...37

Your Action Plan...37

An action plan 37

Ch. 6: Environment Often Matters More Than Motivation, which Is Overrated...........38

Summary 38

Using the environment as a cue...38

Using the complete situation as a cue 39

Key Takeaways from This Chapter 39

Determine Related Issues 39

Your Aspirations...40

Your Strategy 40

Action Plan 40

Ch 7: The Secret of Self-Control 41

Summary 41

Important Takeaways from This Chapter 42

Determine Related Problems...42

Objectives You Want to Reach...42

Your Action Plan...43

An action plan 43

PART THREE: 44

THE 2ND LAW: MAKE IT ATTRACTIVE 44

Ch 8: How to Make a Habit Irresistible 44

Summary 44

Supernormal stimuli..44

Temptations and Dopamine 45

Bundling temptation 45

Principal Takeaways from This Chapter 46

Find Related Issues..46

Objectives You Wish to Achieve 47

Your Strategy for Action...47

Action Checklist..47

Ch. 9: How Your Friends and Family Shape Your Habits....................49

    Summary..49

    The influential members of our society................................49

    The people close to us..49

Important Takeaways from This Chapter................................50

Determine Related Problems..50

Objectives You Want to Reach..51

Your Action Plan..51

An action plan..51

Ch. 10: How to Identify and Address Your Bad Habits' Root Causes..........52

    Summary..52

    the underlying reasons..52

    a change in perspective..53

Important Takeaways from This Chapter................................54

Determine Related Problems..54

Objectives You Want to Reach..54

Your Action Plan..54

An action plan..55

PART FOUR:..56

THE 3RD LAW: MAKE IT EASY..56

Ch 1 1: Walk Slowly, but Never Backward................................56

    Summary..56

    Action versus Motion..56

    How long does it take for new habits to take shape?..................56

Important Takeaways from This Chapter................................57

Determine Related Problems..57

Objectives You Want to Reach..57

Your Action Plan..58

An action plan..58

Ch. 13: The Two-Minute Rule: How to Stop Procrastinating 59

    Summary 59

    Decisions we take 59

    It only takes two minutes.. 59

Important Takeaways from This Chapter 60

Determine Related Problems... 61

Objectives You Want to Reach... 61

Your Action Plan.. 61

An action plan 61

Ch. 14: How to Make Positive Habits Continual and Negative Habits Impossible........... 62

    Summary 62

    Commitment instruments.. 62

Important Takeaways from This Chapter 63

Determine Related Problems... 64

Objectives You Want to Reach... 64

Your Action Plan.. 64

An action plan 64

PART FIVE:.. 65

THE 4TH LAW: MAKE IT SATISFYING 65

Ch. 15: The Fundamental Principle of Behavior Change.............. 65

    Summary 65

Reward types: immediate and delayed 66

Important Takeaways from This Chapter 67

Determine Related Problems... 67

Objectives You Want to Reach... 67

Your Action Plan.. 67

An action plan 67

Ch 16: How to Stick with Good Habits Every Day 69

    Summary 69

    habit monitor 69

Only some people are fans of tracking. 70

What to do if a streak of good habits ends 70

measuring incorrectly 71

Important Takeaways from This Chapter 71

Determine Related Problems.. 71

Objectives You Want to Reach.. 72

Your Action Plan.. 72

An action plan 72

Ch. 17: How a Partner in Accountability Can Transform Everything 73

Summary 73

Habit Agreement... 73

Important Takeaways from This Chapter 74

Determine Related Problems.. 74

Objectives You Want to Reach.. 74

Your Action Plan.. 74

An action plan 74

PART SIX: 76

ADVANCED TACTICS HOW TO GO FROM BEING MERELY GOOD TO BEING TRULY GREAT
.... 76

Ch 18: The Truth About Talent (When Genes Matter and When They Don't)............... 76

Summary 76

Your character and your routine.. 76

Important Takeaways from This Chapter 78

Determine Related Problems.. 78

Objectives You Want to Reach.. 78

Goals you'd like to accomplish... 78

Your Action Plan.. 79

An action plan 79

Chapter 19: The Goldilocks Rule; How to Maintain Motivation at Work and in Life 80

Summary 80

Focusing oneself.. 80

Important Takeaways from This Chapter 81

Determine Related Problems... 81

Objectives You Want to Reach.. 81

your Action Plan... 81

An action plan 82

Ch 20: The Downside of Creating Good Habits............................ 83

Summary.. 83

Important Takeaways from This Chapter 84

Determine Related Problems... 84

Goals You Want to Achieve.. 84

Your Action Plan... 85

An action plan 85

Conclusion:.. 86

The Secret to Results That Last.. 86

INTRODUCTION

James Clear describes being struck in the face with a baseball bat during his sophomore year of high school and the effects of this incident in the prologue to his book.

James's physical problems made it challenging for him to get back to the game he loved. Unfortunately, he was released from the minor league baseball squad.

He finally made it into the college baseball team two years after the accident. But James realized that he needed to be his best self in order to boost his baseball performance and restart his career. At this point, he realized the incredible potential of atomic routines.

James made subtle adjustments, including keeping his room neat, and noticed an increase in his self-assurance. His improved performance in school was the result of new approaches to sleep and study.

He started lifting weights and became a team captain during his junior year of college. Six years after the school accident, he has emerged as one of the best male athletes at Denison. He made the ESPN Academic All-American squad as one of 33 athletes because he consistently built and maintained strong habits. James received the President's Medal, the highest academic accolade, when he graduated.

James acknowledged that he would not have been as successful as he was if he had not dedicated time and effort over time to forming these positive routines and achieving consistent, incremental changes. He was able to recover from his injury and reach his full potential with the adoption of certain simple routines.

As a result, he developed an eagerness to study the science of habit formation and impart his findings to others. Atomic Habits lays out two basic tenets for routine development:

• The "cue-craving-response-reward" paradigm of habit formation.

• How to form useful routines and ditch destructive ones, according to the "four laws of behavior change."

Our habits govern a substantial percentage of our daily activities. Think about brushing your teeth; it's a routine you've done so many times that you probably don't even give it much thought anymore. This is a helpful routine that brings about positive results. Negative, self-defeating habits can grow on autopilot as well. Our poor habits include things like using the snooze button more than once each morning.

Knowing the mechanics of habit formation and how to put that knowledge to use can help you become your greatest self. The purpose of Atomic Habits is to illustrate how altering just one habit may have a profound effect on your life.

In the book's last chapters, James offers a variety of suggestions for maintaining our new routines. The book teaches us a great deal and covers a lot of ground. This guide is meant to make habit development less of a hassle, therefore it covers the most important lessons from the book as well as some significant elements that may have been missed.

PART ONE:

THE FUNDAMENTALS: WHY TINY CHANGES MAKE A BIG DIFFERENCE

CH 1: THE SURPRISING POWER OF ATOMIC HABITS

SUMMARY

In the first section of Atomic Habits, author Tim Ferriss examines how British cycling performance director Dave Brailsford transformed a middling team into an Olympic gold medalist squad in the early 2000s. His method, which he called "the aggregation of marginal gains," was important in this achievement.

MARGINAL GAINS

All aspects of learning to ride a bike were tweaked by the coaching staff by a single percent. For instance, they improved the bike's comfort by redesigning the seats. The fabric of the riders' clothing was upgraded along with the tire grip of the bikes. An orthopedic surgeon was sent in to instruct the bikers on how to properly wash their hands to stave off illness.

Even while each of these adjustments may appear trivial on its own, when taken together they can have a significant impact (known as "marginal gains"). British cyclists won a total of 66 Olympic or Paralympic gold medals, 178 world championships, and 5 Tour de France events in the 5 years after Brailsford began coaching them.

Whence came their success? Brailsford turned around a losing squad by focusing on incremental but meaningful enhancements. Small adjustments can have large effects, as we see here. Brailsford didn't make any major shifts, but he did try to improve upon some minor details.

THE POWER OF 1% CHANGE

While we may believe that "massive success requires massive action," James Clear argues that we "underestimate the value of making small improvements on a daily basis."

Because of their minute size, atoms are invisible to the human sight. However, they are the fundamental components of everything. The sum of these little components, though, can have a profound effect. James Clear calls these imperceptible adjustments (at the atomic level) a 1% boost.

James uses a graph in his book to illustrate how incremental improvements of just 1% per day can yield 37x greater results by the end of the year. If, on the other hand, your condition deteriorates by 1% per day for 365 days, you will end up back at square one.

We must realize that any progress, however small, is preferable to none at all.

But in order to form new, positive routines, the adjustments we make must be maintained over time. Little things add up over time and with repetition. Put another way, excellent habits are like compound interest in that they add up to greater returns over time.

It may take time for the cumulative effect of making little adjustments every day to become apparent. The compound effect can work for both good and negative routines.

Just like you won't be toned after one gym session, you won't see results instantly or even the next day if you consume a bag of snacks for dinner. However, routines pile up with time. You put on weight, usually in the wrong places, from your regular dinner of junk food, and your hard work at the gym shows up in the guise of toned muscles.

The idea behind 1% improvement theory, popularized by James Clear, is that small adjustments can significantly impact and lead to the desired outcomes. A lot of people who try to quit smoking or drinking sugary beverages just give up after a few days because they can't handle the withdrawal symptoms. However, you can achieve your aim of eliminating soft drinks altogether if you gradually lower the number of soft drinks you drink each day. It may take more time, but the benefits will stay far longer.

THE LIMITLESS POTENTIAL PLATEAU

Many people try to form a new, positive habit, but give up when they don't see instant results. If you haven't seen any results yet, James says that doesn't imply they aren't there. There is a plateau of latent Potential that must be broken through before any noticeable change can be seen. It takes time to form a good habit.

When forming a new routine, success is not linear. That is to say, development cannot be mapped out as a straight line from zero to one hundred. Sometimes, transformation occurs when it is invisible to the naked eye. James calls this time the "valley of disappoitment," where many feel like giving up. This is due, in part, to the fact that our culture places a premium on results-oriented actions. It's critical that you go over this point and don't revert back to old ways of behaving.

RESULTS, OBJECTIVES, AND METHODOLOGIES

The outcome or aim is seen by more people as the primary motivator of success. When people are focused solely on the end result, they tend to neglect the steps it takes to get there.

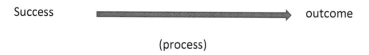

(process)

What accounts for the fact that winners and losers alike strive for the same things but end up with different outcomes? The mechanisms and procedures they've set up hold the key.

When saving for a new car, for instance, winners don't simply save for the car of their dreams; they also improve their long-term savings habits. You will probably reach your objective far more quickly than anticipated if you take this action. Changing your diet will help you lose weight far more quickly than stressing over wearing smaller clothing. According to James Clear, "you fall to the level of your systems rather than the level of your goals."

Instead of focusing just on the end outcome, it is more productive to work toward the adoption of more efficient systems. Your system can be the amount of time you devote to writing each week and the routine you establish in order to achieve your objective, which might be to complete a book. The process (your advancement in the direction of your objective) is driven by your system. Getting what you want requires a systemic approach. Goals (outcomes) help you define a direction, but the processes you put in place are what actually get you where you need to go.

James outlines four issues that arise when you prioritize reaching your goals over developing your infrastructure. This includes:

1. WINNERS AND LOSERS BOTH SHARE THE SAME GOAL

Therefore, the end result is not what sets people apart. It's not enough to simply have a goal in mind if you want to achieve it. Those who succeed do so because they have solid processes in place. Consider the situation of the British cyclists mentioned in the preamble. They, like all the other cyclists, tried to take home the Tour de France trophy each and every year. Everyone was competing to win, but they all went about it in various ways. The British cycling team's success and dominance began after they instituted a system of constant development.

## 2.	A BRIEF CHANGE OCCURS WHEN GOALS ARE ACHIEVED.

A goal being attained causes a brief change. Consider trying to clear up your workspace. You put in that effort one day and succeed in your goal, but if you don't alter the routines or procedures that caused the mess in the first place, you will soon find yourself in the same situation. Alter the systems that lead to the outcomes.

## 3.	GOALS PREVENT YOU FROM BEING HAPPY

Many of us mistakenly believe that if we accomplish our goals, we will be content, and as a result, we keep putting off our happiness until we accomplish those goals or move on to the next. Having a systems-first mentality allows you to enjoy the journey toward your objective. To be happy, you don't have to wait till you accomplish that goal. Your system contains a lot of steps with which you can be satisfied.

## 4.	GOALS DO NOT PROMOTE LONG-TERM ADVANCEMENT.

What occurs when you reach your objective? Do you ever catch yourself falling back into old routines? Having a structure in place will guarantee that you carry on playing the game even after the objective has been met. What happens, for instance, if you reach your optimum weight in relation to your weight loss goal? If you have the right processes in place, they will guarantee that you keep your target weight and stop you from reverting to old behaviors.

You can shift the emphasis away from goals and toward your process by creating a system of atomic habits. Long-term results will be better with a systems-based approach.

Goals = desired outcomes

Systems: are the procedures that lead to the desired outcomes.

IMPORTANT TAKEAWAYS FROM THIS CHAPTER

1. Atomic habits compound, meaning that small adjustments over time accumulate in the same way as compound interest does.

2. We can make significant improvements that endure a lifetime by making minor adjustments to our regular habits.

3. Making little, 1% adjustments over an extended period of time can be more effective than taking massive, singular measures.

4. Rather than focusing only on your goals, you might achieve better results by concentrating on your systems.

5. You can set goals, but don't become so focused on them that you forget about how you're going to get there.

DETERMINE RELATED PROBLEMS

1. Do you have personal goals? Are you constantly certain of the best strategy to accomplish them?

2. Do you start a goal but lose motivation when you don't get results right away?

3. Have you ever experienced disappointment's valley? How did you escape it, exactly?

4. Do you keep track of your development as you work toward your objective?

5. Do you think it's harder to create healthy habits than it is to break bad ones? What makes you believe that is the case?

6. What difficulties did you encounter when attempting to form a new habit?

7. Do you have a defined procedure in place for creating and maintaining new habits?

OBJECTIVES YOU WANT TO REACH

1. I would like to evaluate my present habitual behavior.

2. I want to pinpoint the habits I need to alter or strengthen.

YOUR ACTION PLAN

1. Begin the process of quitting the undesirable behavior and forming the desirable one by:

A. Finding a negative behavior I wish to stop is step one.

B. Finding a positive habit I want to start.

2. Consider the steps you must take to begin forming a beneficial habit or kicking a negative one.

3. Point out any potential roadblocks and try if you can come up with a strategy to get around them.

4. Convince yourself that you can complete the task and succeed. A single forward step is always where change begins. Just take that first step, that's all.

ACTION CHECKLIST

1. Think about your current habits, which ones are productive and which ones are unproductive?

2. Fill in the habit inventory below.

Habit Inventory: Assessing my Habits

What are some of the good habits I already have?	What are some of my bad habits?
	E.g., Eating dessert almost every day
E.g., Saving for my kid's college fund	
What are some good habits I would like to develop?	What are some bad habits I would like to get rid of?

E.g., Drink lemon water every morning   E.g., Cut down on the amount of refined sugar I take in

To help you formulate your thoughts, here are some examples of habits that other people have:

EXAMPLE OF GOOD HABITS:

Healthy eating, exercising regularly, drinking enough water, relaxing, going to bed early, waking up early, cutting down on social media, saving money, decluttering, meditating, practicing a skill, and even making sure to keep in regular contact with people they care about like that weekly phone call to mum.

EXAMPLE OF BAD HABITS:

Overthinking, stressing, eating junk, smoking, watching too much TV, spending too much time on one's phone, procrastinating, overworking, negative thinking, and overspending.

SUMMARY

Good habits are difficult to establish and maintain. James cites two key explanations for this. He claims that we frequently try to alter the wrong thing and that we also approach change in the incorrect way.

In this chapter, we examine the first cause in greater detail: changing the incorrect object.

James identifies three levels at which change can occur to help us comprehend this. He refers to them as the three levels of behavior change.

Results — This is the top layer, where the majority of us start when forming a new habit. Most of the time, we utilize willpower to break bad habits like smoking. The emphasis is on WHAT you hope to accomplish.

Processes is the second layer, which delves a little further. We alter our routines and behaviors, much as when we begin a new fitness program. The HOW of the shift is what is important.

Identity: Of the three layers, this one is the deepest and most internal. Identity is linked to your personality and values. WHO you want to become is the main concern. I might desire to quit smoking or maintain a healthy lifestyle, for instance.

IDENTITY VS. RESULT

Your habits become a part of who you are when you make them a part of your identity.

This encourages you to maintain your practice and make progress toward your objective.

If they wish to change something, the majority of individuals start with the result. For instance, you decide to follow a specific diet in order to lose your belly fat and become healthier (Outcome Identity).

However, if you adopt an identity-based strategy, you might believe: I'm a healthy person, so I'll make sure I eat wholesome foods, drink enough of water, and exercise frequently to lose my belly fat (Identity Outcome).

You'll want to maintain your identity as a healthy person if you truly believe it to be true.

James claims that "true identity change is behavior change." It is more beneficial to start at the identification level rather than the outcome level. When a change becomes a part of who you are, that is the best motivation to make it.

Our behaviors and self-perception are significantly influenced by our beliefs. It is simpler to maintain your new habits over time when they become a part of who you are or who you aspire to be. The only issue with this is that you must watch out for adopting a negative persona, like "I'm a messy person," or something like. That is who I am, period. You are not like that. Ensure your negative behavior is not linked to your identity if you want to change it.

CHANGE WHO YOU ARE TO BENEFIT YOU.

Making change a part of who you are can help you modify your behavior in a real way. A two-step procedure for changing your identity is outlined by James. Choose the kind of person you want to be, and then demonstrate it to yourself by achieving modest victories. You must alter your behavior to alter who you are. For instance, if you want to be a writer, you would tell yourself that you are a writer every time you write something, whether it's a page on your blog or a paragraph in your journal.

Work on being that kind of person if you want to become who you want to be (your identity). Take baby steps to establishing the identity you desire. For instance, I want to be in shape. Ask yourself if a fit person would take the stairs or the elevator when faced with commonplace situations like stairs or elevators at work.

"Your identity shapes your habits, and your habits shape who you are."

IMPORTANT TAKEAWAYS FROM THIS CHAPTER

1. It's difficult to establish excellent habits and maintain them.

2. You must incorporate it into your identity in order to effectively transform your behavior.

3. Habits become a part of who you are when you make them a part of your identity.

4. Your motivation to maintain a habit increases when it becomes a part of who you are.

DETERMINE RELATED PROBLEMS

1. Do you have trouble maintaining a new habit?

2. Do you belong to the group of people who, despite their best efforts, frequently fail to keep their New Year's resolutions?

3. Have you ever taken the time to consider why you struggle to maintain your new routines or resolutions?

4. How long does it often take you to give up new habits?

5. Do you have any habits that have shaped who you are—that is, how you see yourself—in any way?

6. Are you so intent on achieving your goals that you neglect to recognize and appreciate the tiny victories along the way?

OBJECTIVES YOU WANT TO REACH

1. I want to shift my attention from outcomes- to identity-based thinking.

2. I want my new habit to become a permanent part of who I am.

YOUR ACTION PLAN

1. Decide on the new behavior you want to adopt.

2. Create a personal brand that includes your new habit. For instance, because I want to be healthy, I want to start eating more nutritious food and less junk.

3. Make a list of little measures or actions you can take to consistently reinforce your identity statement.

4. Make a list of your behaviors and determine which of them are already a part of who you are. Draw attention to the negative behaviors you want to change, and intentionally incorporate positive traits into your self-identity. For instance, if you wish to break the habit of eating junk food, you may declare that you value health and that eating junk food regularly is not really your thing. Utilize the strength of your self-identity to offer you more motivation as you create healthy habits and stop harmful ones.

AN ACTION PLAN

Think about your aspirations. Consider your interests and core principles. Respond to these inquiries:

1. What kind of outcomes do you hope to achieve? Who is the kind of individual who might succeed in such a situation, you might wonder? Is it, for instance, a person who is dependable or a person who is focused? Concentrate now on those qualities.

2. What aspects of your identity would you alter to suit you better? Instead of concentrating on your goals, think on who you want to become.

SUMMARY

Before moving on, let's examine the science of habit formation in more detail. Our brains store this knowledge when an action is practiced enough to become automatic. as when you brush your teeth. We automatically repeat this action every morning. Our minds create habits.

WHY DO WE DEVELOP ROUTINES?

If we engage in an activity frequently enough, it eventually becomes automatic and is referred to as a habit. When we accomplish an action or behave in a certain way, our brains react by rewarding us. The brain remembers a successful action, whereas a poor effort is forgotten. Through trial and error, our habits are formed.

We attempt something, it fails, we do it again in a new way, it succeeds, we feel happy, we repeat it because it was successful, and after a predetermined number of repetitions, it develops into a habit. The feedback loop that governs human behavior is known as this. We then develop habits based on the behavior we have learned to use to solve difficulties.

The brain no longer has to analyze that specific event in the future for every created habit. This has already happened, and a solution was discovered, so it now happens automatically. Like cleaning your teeth, you are no longer need to think about it. Habits are created through mental shortcuts we've developed over time, freeing our attention for other activities.

HOW CAN WE CREATE HABITS?

James Clear breaks down habit formation into four manageable phases to help people understand how habits function. According to him, all habits go through the following four stages:

CUE

REWARD

CRAVING

RESPONSE

The CUE is what sets off a behavior in our brains. This occurs frequently in reaction to the anticipation of a reward. It could be an object, a particular person, a place, or time.

Craving is what drives us to understand and respond to the cue.

RESPONSE: To state the yearning, we act on the habitual behavior.

REWARD - The response provides us with a bonus of some kind. Every habit has a reward as its eventual objective.

These four steps are repeated in all of our habits. The benefits of sating a craving give us happiness and teach us which behaviors are important to remember. Our habit cycle is completed at this point in the feedback loop. The habit will only develop if all of the four stages are rewarding. Transparent refers to this pattern as the habit loop.

Two phases can be created out of the four steps. While the response and reward are a component of the solution phase, the cue and craving belong to the problem phase. Our actions are typically a response to a particular issue that has to be resolved. To deal with the problems we face, we form habits.

These might be helpful or harmful behaviors if they lead to a solution. If you smoke, for instance, stress at work (trigger) could make you crave going outside to smoke (craving); as a result, you take a quick smoke break (reaction), receive a brief break from the issue at your desk, and enjoy your cigarette (reward).

As a smoker, you have practiced this behavior so frequently that you don't have to think about it. You often feel tempted to go outside and smoke when upset or need a few minutes. It's been ingrained.

Here is another illustration:

You have a paper to write, you need to do some research, you get bored (cue), you feel the urge to amuse yourself (craving), you take out your phone to check social media (reaction), and now you are distracted and engaged (reward). You associate feeling bored with using your phone to check social media. This action is repeated often enough to develop into a habit. When you are bored, you use your phone to pass the time. This may sound familiar to you.

Everything we do is affected by the four stages of cue, craving, reaction, and reward. So, how can we use these four steps to create healthy habits and eliminate harmful ones?

THE FOUR LAWS OF CHANGING BEHAVIOR

The Four Laws of Behavior Change are a collection of straightforward guidelines we may use to form better habits, and they must be considered to establish good practices. James claims that by inverting these laws, we may also use them to break unhealthy habits.

	Good Habits	Bad Habits
Law 1 (Cue)	Make it obvious	Make it Invisible
Law 2 (Craving)	Make it attractive	Make it unattractive
Law 3 (Response)	Make it easy	Make it difficult
Law 4 (Reward)	Make it satisfying	Make it unsatisfying

The secret to eliminating bad habits and forming good ones is this framework. We will explain each of these laws in detail and demonstrate how to apply them in the following section of this worksheet.

IMPORTANT TAKEAWAYS FROM THIS CHAPTER

1. A continuous feedback loop consisting of a cue, a need, a response, and a reward is used to create and reinforce habits.

2. Habits that provide instant gratification are more likely to be continued.

3. To develop a positive habit, make it clear, appealing, simple, and fulfilling.

4. To break a negative habit, make it inconspicuous, unappealing, difficult, and unsatisfying

DETERMINE RELATED PROBLEMS

1. Have you ever given the reasons behind your habits any thought?

2. Which of your habits were consciously created, and which ones are automatic?

3. Are you able to identify with the cue, craving, reaction, and reward loop?

4. Which of your habits stand out the most?

5. Which of your habits makes you feel the happiest?

OBJECTIVES YOU WANT TO REACH

1.1 I want to know why I do the things I do and how to develop healthier habits.

2.2 I want to be able to methodically break any harmful habits I may have by having a better understanding of the habit loop and the 4 rules of behavior modification.

YOUR ACTION PLAN

1. Decide on a few habits I wish to start or change, or at least two.

2. I'll categorize them in accordance with the stages of the habit loop to help you better comprehend my habitual behavior.

3. Consider your habits in the context of the habit loop for a moment. It might be able to offer insightful information on your habit formation and triggers.

ACTION CHECKLIST

1.   Make a list of habits you would like to work on.

2.   Take one of your good habits and put them through the habit cycle like in the smoking example and the writing example given earlier on in this chapter. Use this template to assist you:

Habita	CUE	CRAVING	RESPONSE	REWARD
Good Habits				

Habits	CUE	CRAVING	RESPONSE	REWARD

Bad Habits:

Habits   CUE   CRAVING   RESPONSE   REWARD

Good Habits

Habits   CUE   CRAVING   RESPONSE   REWARD

Bad Habit

SUMMARY

Make it evident, that the first rule of behavior modification addresses the cue stage of habit building. The cue is what prompts you to carry out your habit. You must be clear about a new practice you want to develop.

Our brains are remarkably adept at detecting pertinent clues in a variety of circumstances. According to James, this skill is the basis for our habit. We do so many things without giving them a second thought. Because of this, we may miss the indication that signals the beginning of a habit.

It's not always a good thing when we develop habits without realizing it, especially when such habits turn out to be harmful ones. Because of this, James says that starting with awareness is crucial when creating a new habit. If we are conscious that we have a habit in the first place, we can only work to change it.

JAMES OFFERS TWO METHODS WE MIGHT DO TO BECOME MORE CONSCIOUS OF OUR HABITS:

• **Pointing-and-Calling:** A method for making an unconscious habit more visible by increasing awareness. For instance, you might list everything you need before leaving the house in the morning, such as your phone, briefcase, car keys, etc. This will help you remember everything.

You can use the Habits Scorecard activity to increase your awareness of your habit. It is required to make a list of your regular behaviors and mark them with a plus sign (+) for positive behaviors or a minus sign (-) for negative behaviors. A =(equal) symbol can represent a neutral habit. When evaluating your habits, consider their long-term value and whether they support or contradict your desired identity.

- **The habits scorecard** should be completed since it will help you become more conscious of which behaviors are good for you and which are bad.

IMPORTANT TAKEAWAYS FROM THIS CHAPTER

1. Make it clear that you want to develop good habits.

2. Automatic habit formation is not always desirable, mainly when we develop negative habits.

3. You must be conscious of having a habit before you can change, improve, or eliminate it.

4. There are two methods we might employ to increase awareness of our habits: Pointing, calling, and a scorecard for your habits

IDENTIFY RELATED ISSUES

1. Do you know all of your good and evil habits?

2. Do you believe that becoming conscious of your behaviors will be helpful in any way?

3. How do you believe awareness can assist you in changing your ingrained behaviors?

OBJECTIVES YOU WANT TO REACH

1. I wish to pay closer attention to my routines.

2. I wish to increase my awareness of my habits using the two awareness approaches.

YOUR ACTION PLAN

1. Use the point-and-call method When you leave the house tomorrow or after work. If you're employing the approach for the first time, go slowly. Concentrate on the main points that you find essential. Gradually broaden the list as you continue to use the strategy and notice your situational awareness improving.

2. Completing the Habits Scorecard.

AN ACTION PLAN

1. What have you learned about the point-and-call method?

2. Write down all of your daily routines, starting when you get up and ending when you go to bed. Once you've finished making your list, go through it and indicate which habits you think are good (with a plus sign (+)) and which you believe are harmful (with a minus sign (-)). Mark something with a (=) if you need to know whether it's good or terrible. Lists can be created using the template below.

Habits Rating Scale

My Daily Habits	Good +	Bad -	Neutral =

Note: A good habit is usually one that helps you to reinforce your desired identity or helps you become the type of person you wish to be. Bad habits are usually the ones that conflict with who you want to be.

CH 5: THE BEST WAY TO START A NEW HABIT

SUMMARY

The easiest method to begin a new habit is to make an intentional strategy in advance. You'll be more likely to achieve your goals if you have a detailed strategy outlining how to execute your new habit. James refers to this kind of plan as an implementation aim.

APPLICATION OBJECTIVE

Time and place are the two most typical triggers that can start a habit. The likelihood that you will follow through on the plan is increased if you describe your habit in terms of an implementation intention and include the time and location.

Saying I'll [Action - do this] at [this time] in [this area], for instance, would be a firmer commitment. Clarifying the specifics of when and where you will carry out the activity makes your goal more evident than making a general statement like, "I will exercise more" or "I will practice the piano more."

One statement can serve as an implementation strategy for a particular activity or behavior, for example:

At six in the morning, I'll stretch out on my patio.

Or

I'll go for a power walk with my partner in our neighborhood at 5 o'clock.

We accomplish our goals more frequently when we are clear about what we want to achieve, when we will do it, and how we will do it. Making ambiguous promises, such as I'll start working out tomorrow, makes it simpler to put something off. With the help of an implementation strategy, you can practice your behavior until it becomes automatic and second nature.

According to James, there are numerous methods for us to apply implementation intents in our daily lives. His main technique is habit stacking. We frequently base a lot of our decisions on what we just finished doing. For instance, washing the dishes may prompt the memory to soak the dishtowels for subsequent washing. You might then be reminded to load the washer, which might prompt you to put a softener on your shopping list, and so on. Every action you take has the potential to serve as a cue for a subsequent action. The reason for this is that "no behavior happens in isolation."

HABIT-STACKING

The next step is to choose an existing habit to build your new habit on top of. As an illustration, following [CURRENT HABITI, 1 will [NEW HABIT I. This technique, named the habit stacking formula by James, was created by BJ Fogg.

Your new habit is sparked by your present one.

An illustration of habit stacking is as follows:

I want to start meditating every day as a new habit.

Habit accumulation: I meditate for 90 seconds every morning after brewing my coffee.

Making your desired behavior dependent on an everyday habit you currently have can help you maintain your new habit. Once you get used to it, you can combine a number of tiny habits.

James gives a good illustration of how this might function:

1. I'll meditate for 60 seconds after making my morning coffee.

2. I'll make my to-do list for the day after a 60-second meditation.

3. I will get started on my first task right away after writing my daily to-do list.

He also offers a straightforward illustration of how you might incorporate your new habit into your old routine:

Currently, I get up, make my bed, and then take a shower.

Extended routine: Make my bed, lay a book on my pillow, then get ready for the shower.

My new nightly routine now includes reading a few pages of my book. Your book is ready for you when you climb into bed at night.

You need the correct cue to get things started to build a successful habit stack. Some new habits could not be compatible with your current routines because of the wrong occasion or environment. The best course of action is to review your list of daily routines, then figure out where and how to incorporate your new desired habit into your current routine. Just make sure you are clear about the information and not ambiguous.

Making your behavior change clear (i.e., the first law of behavior change) is facilitated by techniques like implementation goals and habit stacking.

IMPORTANT TAKEAWAYS FROM THIS CHAPTER

1. Describe your new habit's implementation in detail. Be clear about what you want to achieve.

2. You can lay out your new habit's implementation strategy with an implementation plan.

3. The time and place are two cues that can start a habit. Add them to your strategy.

4. behavior stacking, which involves combining two habits, makes it easier to incorporate a new behavior into an existing routine.

DETERMINE RELATED PROBLEMS

1. When attempting to form a good habit, are you clear about your goals?

2. How precisely will you implement it?

3. Do you find it challenging to incorporate a new habit into your daily routine?

4. Do you believe habit stacking will be successful for you?

5. Which two behaviors may you combine?

OBJECTIVES YOU WANT TO REACH

1.1 I want to implement my new behaviors deliberately and precisely.

2. I want to incorporate my new habits into my daily activities.

YOUR ACTION PLAN

1. Create an implementation plan.

2. Use habit stacking, or adding a new habit on top of an existing one.

AN ACTION PLAN

1. Create a few implementation goals for your new routines, like these:

At [add the time here] in [add the location here], I will [add what you will do here].

2. Apply habit stacking: I'll start [new behavior] after [current habit]. See where and how you might incorporate your new desired habit into your everyday schedule after reviewing your list of daily routines. For instance:

3. Behavior stacking, or adding a new behavior to an existing one, will make the habit (go to the gym) noticeable. Add going to the gym on top of your routine of getting into your car at work to head home. When you get into your car (cue), drive to the gym rather than your house.

SUMMARY

Human conduct is greatly influenced by the environment.

James tells a tale of an experiment in which the chief medical officer of a hospital in Boston made the decision to alter the cafeteria's design in an effort to affect the eating habits of the hospital workers. In refrigerators near to the cash registers that had previously only stored soda, researchers put water. Additionally, strategically placed baskets of bottled water were scattered throughout the cafeteria. Nothing about this was communicated to the personnel.

The hospital cafeteria's soda sales decreased during the ensuing several months, while bottled water sales began to increase, according to researchers. When they changed the meals to be healthier, the outcomes remained the same. This experiment demonstrates that people frequently decide based on where options are rather than what they are.

We develop habits mostly as a result of our environment. Every habit is context-dependent, according to James. We frequently act or make decisions depending on what we observe or other visual signals.

USING THE ENVIRONMENT AS A CUE

We can use our environment to set off a habit because every habit is started by a signal. We can alter our surroundings to make a cue more clear. For instance, I'd want to go for a stroll every day at 5:00 PM. In this case, time serves as a trigger to get you to start the action. You can also build your surroundings around this time-triggered action to reinforce it. For instance, if you put on your walking clothes or shoes as soon as you get home from work, you are more likely to stick to your routine and not make an excuse or put it off till later and then not do it. Additionally, you can make sure they are kept in a location where you cannot avoid seeing them.

There will be fewer steps between you and the ideal conduct and more between you and the undesirable behavior as a result.

If you want to enhance your exposure to positive cues, you can scatter triggers around your environment. For instance, you might need to increase the amount of water you consume each day. You can keep a bottle of water on your desk and another on the

kitchen counter so that you can notice it as soon as you enter the room. One can be left on your nightstand as a reminder to drink water when you wake up.

USING THE COMPLETE SITUATION AS A CUE

A habit may be triggered by a specific stimulus on occasion or by the environment you are in other times. There may be multiple triggers present at once. By tying a behavior to a particular setting, a habit can be formed. According to James, it is simpler to reinforce a new habit in an unfamiliar environment than in one with familiar environmental cues. For instance, if you wish to stop smoking, avoid going to the neighborhood bar where everyone is smoking (at least until your new habit takes hold).

Create a new environment, relocate, or change your current environment to accommodate your new habit. It is simpler to create and maintain a habit when it has a defined and consistent surroundings.

KEY TAKEAWAYS FROM THIS CHAPTER

1. Our habits and behaviors can be significantly influenced by our environment.

2. We frequently base our decisions on the visual cues we see around us.

3. Environmental cues like time and place can support the development of new habits.

4. By connecting a particular behavior to a particular setting, it can be developed.

DETERMINE RELATED ISSUES

1. Do you notice that you pick up behaviors from the environment around you?

2. Do you believe that occasionally, you unintentionally adopt the routines of those around you?

3. Which of your present behaviours have been influenced by your surroundings?

4. Which of your present behaviors are simpler to keep up since you've changed your surroundings to facilitate them?

5. Do you want to start a new habit that you believe will be aided by environmental cues?

6. Is your environment set up in a way that makes it simple to practice your habit?

7. What would you alter in your surroundings to make it more beneficial for you?

YOUR ASPIRATIONS

1. In order to better support my habits, I will alter or rearrange my environment.

2. I'll make it easier to recognize the signs of healthy habits.

YOUR STRATEGY

1. Change your surroundings to make your behavior more visible. Would you like to hydrate yourself more? Fill some water bottles, then scatter them throughout your home, paying particular attention to high traffic areas.

2. When establishing new habits or breaking bad ones, be mindful of where you travel. Create a mobility plan for your day to identify any surroundings that can prevent you from forming new habits and then come up with a solution.

ACTION PLAN

1. Recognize your environmental cues and make use of them. Time and place are the two most potent triggers.

2. Using time and/or place, write down your purpose. For instance:

Time: I exercise first thing in the morning on Saturdays or I work out. My desk at home or the gym.

SUMMARY

Research on drug addictions conducted in the 1970s by Lee Robins demonstrated that a drastic shift in the surrounding circumstances could result in the cessation of an obsession. Sometimes, a negative behavior persists just because one is constantly exposed to factors that cause it. The habit vanishes when the cues are removed, or the environment is altered. This demonstrates how a habit can alter depending on the context.

The findings of Robins' study also demonstrated that some people only sometimes adhere to their habits due to a lack of self-control. Self-control can be aided by establishing a more structured atmosphere. You can break a harmful habit by removing the clues from your surroundings.

We are all aware that poor habits are challenging to break. According to studies, even after a habit has been ingrained in your memory and you may believe you have kicked it to the curb, contextual cues can cause you to pick it back up. James uses the example of smoking to demonstrate this.

She lit a cigarette every time Patty Olwell rode horseback with a buddy. Years later, when she had stopped riding horses and had quit smoking, she found herself back on a horse. This time, the need to smoke came on effortlessly. She was not inclined to smoke because she had not been exposed to environmental cues like horseback riding. Therefore, even if you can break a problematic behavior, you might still remember it.

Your environment can provide cues that encourage you to repeat a poor behavior. "Cueinduced wanting" is the term for this. Most of the time, we are not consciously aware of it. As in Chapter 6's illustration of smoking in a bar.

James claims that cutting off a harmful habit at the source is one of the finest methods to eliminate it. An inversion of the first law of behavior modification is to reduce exposure to the stimulus that triggers the habit. The cue is not made evident; instead, it is made invisible.

Since self-control is a short-term tactic, eliminating the cue might be a better long-term solution to break a harmful habit.

For instance, if your phone keeps ringing while you're working and you can't stop answering it, put it in another room. You won't become distracted from your job if it doesn't beep every time a notice comes in. Another illustration is to transfer the TV from the bedroom to another room if you discover that you watch too much TV right before bed.

Sometimes, all it takes to break a habit is a minor adjustment. If the cue is gone, you won't be lured by it. Make it undetectable. By limiting your exposure to the things that cause harmful behaviors, you can get rid of them.

IMPORTANT TAKEAWAYS FROM THIS CHAPTER

1. The first law of behavior modification, "make it obvious," is inverted to "make it invisible."

2. Environmental cues can encourage you to continue a harmful habit.

3. Make a harmful habit invisible to help you break it.

4. Limit your time in settings or circumstances that could tempt you.

DETERMINE RELATED PROBLEMS

1. Do you find yourself adopting bad habits from the context around you?

2. Which of your current bad habits are formed by your environment?

3. Is there a bad habit you want to give up where you think environmental cues would help?

4. Is your environment designed so that your habit is harder to act on?

5. What will you change in your environment to better serve you?

OBJECTIVES YOU WANT TO REACH

1. I will rebuild or reorganize my environment to support my strategy to break my harmful habit.

2. Make my harmful habit's triggers invisible.

YOUR ACTION PLAN

1. Increase my awareness of my surroundings to determine if there are any indicators I can eliminate that support my harmful habit.

2. Remove environmental cues from my poor behaviors to lessen exposure.

3. It would be helpful to use the situational awareness and mindfulness you have been working on to assist you in identifying the environmental signals that cause your habits in this section. Always remember that being more aware of your surroundings is a positive and beneficial thing.

AN ACTION PLAN

1. Decide which harmful habits you can eliminate by eliminating environmental triggers. Making the cues undetectable. Put your implementation goals in writing, like this:

I will steer clear of the grocery store's junk food department as part of my effort to cut back on [for example, junk food].

OR

I'll stop purchasing junk food to keep at home as part of my effort to cut back on it.

CH 8: HOW TO MAKE A HABIT IRRESISTIBLE

SUMMARY

In the second section of the workbook, we look at how to make a habit appealing enough to motivate us to keep it up. Making a habit attractive is the first aspect of the 2nd Law of Behavior Change, which is covered in this chapter on how to make a habit irresistible.

SUPERNORMAL STIMULI

Exaggerated cues are what scientists refer to as supernormal stimuli. As humans, we are frequently susceptible to this kind of stimuli. We tend to crave them because we typically see them as rewards. Foods heavy in sugar, salt, or fat are a good example of junk food. Products with high quantities of these components are frequently presented in appealing packaging to draw in customers.

Food manufacturers take use of the fact that we consume more of it when it is appealing to our senses, tasty, and appealing to our eyes and tastes. Businesses invest a lot of time and money in research to ensure that processed meals have unique flavors or textures that natural foods do not, in an effort to increase the consumption of those items. According to James, this is a good illustration of the second law of behavior change, which states that you should make something appealing. Something has a higher chance of developing a habit if it is more enticing.

Businesses, advertising, and social media platforms sometimes inflate information about things besides food. Everything in our world, from altered photographs to advertisements, has an inflated reality. We are continuously inundated with alluring stimuli and incentives. So it seems to reason that in order to make our behaviors desirable to us, we need make them irresistible.

TEMPTATIONS AND DOPAMINE

Knowing more about cravings and how they function can help us better grasp how to make a habit impossible to avoid. Researchers found that the neurotransmitter dopamine was the cause of our appetites and desires for particular behaviors and goods while conducting an experiment.

When you feel pleasure or receive a reward, the chemical dopamine is released in the brain. According to James, routines constitute a "dopamine-driven feedback loop." To put it another way, when you enjoy yourself, your dopamine levels rise, and as your dopamine levels rise, your urge to act likewise rises.

You are motivated to behave when you are anticipating a reward. Your dopamine level increases when you either obtain or expect a reward. As a result, when you receive a reward for the first time when acquiring a new behavior, dopamine is produced. In anticipation of the reward the following time, dopamine is also released. Dopamine is released in anticipation as soon as your brain identifies the cue for the habit. When you perceive a trigger after learning a habit and don't respond to it, there is no reward and your dopamine levels fall.

This demonstrates to us how wanting and desire play a significant influence in our habitual behavior. Because the hope of receiving a reward encourages us to behave, we must thus make our routines appealing. James provides what he calls temptation packaging as a tactic to capitalize on this.

BUNDLING TEMPTATION

This tactic functions by connecting a desired action with a required action. For instance, I might watch TV as I run on the treadmill because I need to keep up my workout routine but I also want to watch TV.

The craving component of the habit loop is connected to this kind of behavior. Making habits appealing will aid in their maintenance. We begin linking the reward with the cue. In anticipation of viewing my favorite show, getting on the treadmill becomes more appealing.

To achieve even greater success, temptation bundling and habit stacking (chapter 5) might be combined:

Stacking habits: After (current habit), I'll do (needed habit).

Combining temptations: After (habit I need), I'll do (habit I want).

Example:

I'll stretch (if necessary) after drinking my morning coffee.

I'll read the book I want to read after I stretch.

By fulfilling your obligations, such as reading your book, you are able to achieve your goals. Habit formation is more alluring when temptation is bundled.

PRINCIPAL TAKEAWAYS FROM THIS CHAPTER

1. Make a good habit enticing if you want to develop it.

2. Advertisements frequently use exaggerated cues to pique our interest in us as people.

3. Our desires and rewards cycle are caused by the neurotransmitter dopamine.

4. One strategy for making a habit appealing is to utilize cues (rewards) to make it alluring.

5. Make your habit more appealing to encourage you to remain with it by using temptation bundling.

FIND RELATED ISSUES

1. Do you ever get hungry?

2. What are your cravings—both good and bad—right now?

3. What do you do in the presence of cravings?

4. Do you give in to every craving?

5. Have you ever had a need for something because of too dramatic stimuli in your environment?

6. Are you aware of the underlying causes of your cravings?

OBJECTIVES YOU WISH TO ACHIEVE

1. I want to be able to identify the need that fuels my addiction.

2. I want to leverage my urges to make my healthy habit impossible to resist.

YOUR STRATEGY FOR ACTION

1. Recognize my cravings and the driving force behind them.

2. Use a temptation bundling strategy and combine it with habit stacking to be more effective.

ACTION CHECKLIST

1.   Identify and make a list of your cravings.

Next to each craving write down what you think is the deeper underlying motivation for each craving. For example, I crave salty snacks because they comfort me when I am feeling down or I crave buying more books because reading helps me to relieve boredom/learn new things.

Use the template below

What is my craving?   Why do I crave this?

2.		Use temptation bundling with or without habits stacking. Pair an action you want to do with an action you need to do. For example, I will do my morning stretches while I catch up on an episode of my favorite musical piece while I go on my 30 minute jog.

CH. 9: HOW YOUR FRIENDS AND FAMILY SHAPE YOUR HABITS

SUMMARY

Your habits are also influenced by the people you spend time with. This is especially true regarding your friends and family, who are the closest to you.

Your behavior is influenced by the habits of the people around you and by your culture. Your early patterns were probably created due to watching others replicate conduct. We are only sometimes conscious of how our behavior is influenced by the social norms we are exposed to as children.

We frequently adopt other people's habits to blend in. According to James, we frequently adopt the behaviors of three different social groups: those close to us, those we interact with often, and those who hold positions of authority. These people's actions may make it more appealing for us to adopt certain habits. Keep in mind that the second law of behavior change is attraction.

THE INFLUENTIAL MEMBERS OF OUR SOCIETY

One group that encourages us to break a habit is "the powerful." Power, status, and actions that earn approval and respect are all things that humans are drawn to. We desire to stand out once we have assimilated into a group. As a result, we turn to the behaviors of successful people or those we respect. We attempt to act similarly to them. We are drawn to actions that earn us respect, admiration, and status.

THE PEOPLE CLOSE TO US

We mimic or adopt the habits of those who are close to us. And occasionally, we act in this way without even realizing it. You begin speaking in the other person's voice or adopting their stance. According to one study, the partner of someone who loses weight in a relationship is very likely to follow suit.

Joining a community or culture where the behavior you want to exhibit (i.e., the habit you want to acquire) is accepted behavior, according to James, is an excellent approach to develop healthier habits. For instance, you are more likely to desire to exercise and get fitter if you want to be fit and hang out with other fit individuals. You're more likely to succeed as a group if you hang out with people who want to form the same habits as you.

Even better, if you can find your tribe—people who are like you or who share your interests—and they share the same drive, your individual quest will become one that the entire tribe is on. Anything from a reading club to a band might be your tribe. Not only can you all get up at once, but by sticking with the group even after your objectives have been met, you are more likely to find it simpler to continue your habits.

Groups control our conduct when we are unsure how to behave. We scan the area to see what everyone is up to. The drawback to this is that if you need to change a habit that goes against the grain of the tribe, you could fear that you won't fit in and this might make the new habit less appealing. Only when a change puts you in your place will it be appealing?

IMPORTANT TAKEAWAYS FROM THIS CHAPTER

1. Make a good habit appealing to develop it.

2. We are frequently pulled to the societal norms of others around us.

3. At times, we copy other people's actions to fit in with a group or to model ourselves after strong people we look up to.

4. It can be simpler to keep up a new habit when you meet people who have similar tendencies to you.

5. The drawback is that you can be hesitant to break a poor habit because it is ingrained in your society and you don't want to stand out by deviating from the norm.

DETERMINE RELATED PROBLEMS

1. Do you believe you may have inherited any tendencies from your close friends or family members?

2. Do you believe you have acquired any behaviors from any influential people in society whom you admire?

3. Do you belong to any communities that share your habits?

4. Would you join a group that emphasized a brand-new habit you were beginning?

5. Do you believe that becoming a part of this kind of group would inspire you to maintain your routine?

6. What happens if the group no longer abides by your new constructive behavior? Do you want to stay or go?

OBJECTIVES YOU WANT TO REACH

1. I want to ensure that my new habit is compelling enough to continue.

2. I want to locate a group that can assist me in keeping up my new habit.

YOUR ACTION PLAN

1. Join a group ("culture") where your preferred habit is accepted as the standard.

2. Try to avoid or distance yourself from any groups that are encouraging bad habits that you want to change.

AN ACTION PLAN

1. Look up an organization you can join online by doing some investigation.

Or

Find out if any local organizations share your interests. Discover how to sign up as a member.

2. After being a part of your group for a few weeks or months, return to this area and respond to the following questions:

a. Do you think being a part of the group makes it easier for you to keep up your new habit?

b. How does it benefit you? For instance, are the successes and failures of the other group members inspiring to you? Do you learn from their mistakes? Do you get support and encouragement from being a part of the group?

c. Will you stick with the group even after effectively ingraining your positive habit into your identity? Why?

CH. 10: HOW TO IDENTIFY AND ADDRESS YOUR BAD HABITS' ROOT CAUSES

SUMMARY

The second law of behavior change, "make it attractive," was discussed in detail in the first two chapters. This chapter examines the reverse of this law, which is to make something undesirable.

Making a harmful habit ugly will make it more likely that you will stop doing it.

THE UNDERLYING REASONS

Let's start by considering where our appetites initially originate. Every hunger typically has a deeper cause. things like obtaining food or water, making connections with others, winning others' favor, and so forth. Most habit-forming items don't inspire fresh enthusiasm. Instead, they arouse cravings by appealing to human nature's deeper desires.

For instance, our basic desire to connect and form bonds with others is the root of the habit of monitoring social media. Uncertain of a fact? We look for information on Google in order to achieve the overarching goal of eliminating ambiguity. We develop habits based on our fundamental human impulses. These have remained constant throughout history.

However, there are other strategies to address underlying reasons. For instance, one individual may find that going for a run helps them relax, while another person may find that going outside for a smoke does. By doing this, you are linking your behavior to a problem. You have an issue, which your habit deals with and resolves in this manner. I'm stressed; I'll de-stress by running; or I'm stressed; I'll de-stress by smoking.

Constant correlations and predictions are made by our brains. This will occur if we take this action. I'm going to eat this ice cream gently because if I eat it too quickly, I'll get brain freeze. Our behaviors and routines are heavily influenced by the predictions we make. They also depend on how each person perceives the world (how we see things). Someone else could believe that if I don't consume this ice cream quickly, it will melt in the heat and drip all over me.

As a result, the same trigger might lead to either a positive or negative habit. And this is based on how you feel and what you anticipate will happen. Our emotions guide our decisions regarding whether or not to change anything. We find habits that are connected

to pleasant emotions more appealing. We get a yearning to repeat a behavior when it successfully addresses an underlying reason.

A CHANGE IN PERSPECTIVE

We need to correlate difficult behaviors with satisfying experiences in order to make them more appealing to us. According to James, we may rewire our brains to choose challenging behaviors. Here's where just a small mental adjustment can be beneficial. For instance, changing the word "have" to "get" creates a significant difference in how you see a challenging habit.

You might say I GET to write another chapter as opposed to I HAVE to write another chapter. You are allowed to go to the gym and make your bed. While you must perform these tasks, you also have the option to do so. With this mentality change, these things become possibilities rather than burdens or tasks.

Your habits become more appealing when you reframe them to emphasize their advantages. For instance, you can view saving money as the future financial independence you will have rather than as a sacrifice you must make.

James advises you to take this a step further by developing a motivation routine. To put it another way, try linking your habits to enjoyable activities so that you may use that cue whenever you need a little boost of motivation. James gives a nice illustration of how he applied a similar technique to put himself in the correct frame of mind to perform before a game:

I had a set routine for stretching and throwing before every game throughout my time playing baseball. The entire process took me ten minutes, and I followed the identical steps each and every time. It got me physically ready to play, but more significantly, it got me mentally prepared. I started to link my pre-game routine with having a competitive and focused mindset. Even if I hadn't been inspired before, by the time my routine was over, I was in "game mode."

By changing the associations you have with your harmful habits, you can eliminate their root causes. Think about the reasons behind your negative behaviours. Use this to your advantage by making them unappealing and the trigger for a good habit more alluring.

IMPORTANT TAKEAWAYS FROM THIS CHAPTER

1. Make a bad habit unattractive to get rid of it.

2. There is frequently an underlying motivation behind the habits we develop.

3. Determining the underlying motivation can assist us in transforming a poor habit into a positive one.

4. The same cues can result in either a healthy habit or a poor habit.

5. Reframe your relationship with your harmful habit to make it less alluring.

DETERMINE RELATED PROBLEMS

1. Review your habit scorecard's list of undesirable behaviors once more. Why did you call those negative behaviors?

2. Consider the reasons behind how you came to form those habits in the first place. Was there a hidden reason behind this terrible habit?

3. How can you use constructive connections or cues to assist you break undesirable habits?

OBJECTIVES YOU WANT TO REACH

1. I wish to lessen the allure of my unhealthy habits.

2. A methodical approach to kicking undesirable behaviors would be ideal.

YOUR ACTION PLAN

1. To change your poor behaviors into good ones, use the reasons behind them.

2. Realize the advantages of quitting your undesirable habits.

3. Keep a journal of your wants and urges so you can track whether ones are linked to good or unhealthy habits.

AN ACTION PLAN

1. Recognize the reasons why you began your bad behaviours. What wants or desires caused them?

2. Describe the advantages of kicking your undesirable behaviors in writing.

3. List the ways in which you might lessen the appeal of each of your negative habits.

PART FOUR:

THE 3RD LAW: MAKE IT EASY

CH 1 1: WALK SLOWLY, BUT NEVER BACKWARD

SUMMARY

Sometimes, when we want to alter anything in our lives, it's easy to become overwhelmed by the logistics. We spend so much time determining the optimal course of action that we never actually carry out the plan.

ACTION VERSUS MOTION

We must understand that motion and action are not the same thing. Sometimes, even though we believe we are acting (planning, acquiring knowledge, and strategizing), we are actually in motion. Results are not produced by activity; they are made by acts.

For example, if you decide to switch to a better eating plan, you would make that decision by conducting all the necessary research and planning. The activity is to sit down and cook and eat that nutritious meal.

We are acting and moving forward when there is motion in a shift. Being active is simple, but progress is impeded when procrastination replaces planning and preparation. According to James, rather than meticulous planning, repetition and practice work best when establishing new habits. Make it simple, says the third law.

HOW LONG DOES IT TAKE FOR NEW HABITS TO TAKE SHAPE?

As previously stated, habits form when behaviors are repeated frequently enough. Repeating behaviors cause specific brain regions to change, according to scientists. Like the muscles in our bodies, they respond to changes more readily the more we use them. Actively practicing a recurring activity increases success since the brain starts to carry it out automatically.

As a result, habits don't require as much focus after a few repetitions. They turn automatic after they cross what Clear refers to as "the habit line". We carry out the acts automatically, and a new habit is created. According to studies, habit formation is based more on frequency than time.

Many people are curious about the length of time it takes to form a new habit, but Clear argues that this is the wrong question to pose because habits are formed through repetition. How many repetitions would it take to create an automatic habit? Might be a better question.

Your hit rate—the number of times you try the new activity successfully—determines whether you'll develop a habit. After several successful attempts, the new behavior solidifies in your brain, and you cross the habit threshold.

IMPORTANT TAKEAWAYS FROM THIS CHAPTER

1. Sometimes, preparation gives us the impression that we are moving forward.

2. Planning is a process; it does not result in results.

3. We must act and take action to see results.

4. Avoid spending too much time planning and forgetting to start.

5. Repetitions develop habits; performance rate matters more than required training time.

DETERMINE RELATED PROBLEMS

1. Do you tend to put things off? Do you need to work on tasks you intend to complete?

2. Do you develop complex plans but fail to carry them out?

3. Do you prefer to jump right into the action-oriented aspect?

4. Do you care more about the length of time it will take you to develop your new habit?

5. Are you aware that repetitions rather than the time spent doing something help create habits?

OBJECTIVES YOU WANT TO REACH

1. I want to act on my goals and see them through.

2. I want to successfully repeat my new behavior until I cross the habit threshold to ingrain it.

YOUR ACTION PLAN

1. Conduct the necessary research, make your plans, and carry them out.

2. Begin my new routine.

3. Continue practicing my new behavior until it is deeply ingrained in my brain.

AN ACTION PLAN

1. Pick a behavior you wish to start as soon as possible from your habits scorecard, such as reading a book or consuming low-carb meals.

2. Set a start date on your calendar and resolve to begin.

3. Take a couple of days to complete any necessary planning, purchasing, or research.

4. Begin the habit on your start date and maintain it daily until it is ingrained in your behavior. Utilize the ideas and approaches you have already learned about in the chapters before to help you.

CH. 13: THE TWO-MINUTE RULE: HOW TO STOP PROCRASTINATING

SUMMARY

The two-minute rule is another method James discusses for making habits more straightforward. This chapter explores the two-minute rule's anti-procrastination benefits, which are especially helpful for habitual procrastinators.

We are aware that a sizable amount of our daily activities are habit-driven. But more than that, those routines also have a significant impact on the judgments and choices we make. Some behaviors may take a few seconds to perform, yet they may have a more significant impact on our future behavior.

DECISIONS WE TAKE

We have "decisive moments" where we must make decisions every day. For instance, if you walk to your car after work and pass a restaurant serving takeout, that split-second when deciding whether to order takeout or make supper at home is your pivotal one.

Every decision we make at these critical times is similar to a fork in the road. They accumulate during the day and produce various results. There are multiple possibilities at the takeaway you were passing. According to James, you are now in charge of what you order, but your selections are just those they offer.

Similarly, we are constrained by our ingrained decision directions. Understanding that our habits are just the beginning of our journey when we start building new ones is crucial. Creating little is preferable to starting large. When making a change, the two-minute rule enables you to start modestly rather than attempting to do too much too fast.

IT ONLY TAKES TWO MINUTES.

Making a habit simpler to start by scaling it down to a two-minute version. Consider the scenario where you want to begin a new tradition of reading each night before bed, but you keep putting it off. Once you get going, continuing will be simpler, so start with only one page. Read three pages the following night, and so on. The new habit will be easy if the initial two minutes are simple. The acts might get harder and produce more results as the habit develops.

James refers to this simple two-minute start as the "gateway" habit. Gateway behaviors let you progress from extremely simple to challenging, ultimately leading to the desired result. Let's examine how it functions using the reading example from earlier.

Reading every night before going to sleep.

Very	Easy	Moderate	Hard	Very Hard
Reading 1 page	Reading 4 page	Reading 1 chapter	Reading 6 Chapters	Reading the Entire book

The example here is relatively straightforward yet effectively illustrates the principle. The important thing is to start and take essential action. If you develop the habit of showing up, you can create the habit by regularly performing simple tasks before developing the skill and tackling the more complex tasks.

The initial two minutes of your process of breaking an old habit or creating a new one serve as a ritual. It resembles warming up before an exercise in many ways. Making the initial action effortless to initiate frequently encourages the rest to flow. The two-minute rule requires little commitment, making it simple to establish as a habit. After two minutes, put down the book. If you do it this way, reading won't seem like something you have to do.

The two-minute rule, in conjunction with a habit-shaping strategy, can assist you in advancing your habit toward your desired outcome. Learn how to do your two-minute action in its simplest form. Pick a book, place it on your pillow in the morning, remove it when you go to bed, and read for one minute, 90 seconds, and two minutes. You will eventually be able to mold your reading habit to fit your intention to read every night before you sleep.

IMPORTANT TAKEAWAYS FROM THIS CHAPTER

1. Daily decisions that we make set us on our habitual course.

2. Apply the two-minute rule to break bad habits and stop procrastinating.

3. Molding a new habit following our aims can be done in as little as two minutes.

4. Begin with your gateway habit and gradually up the difficulty of your difficulties.

DETERMINE RELATED PROBLEMS

1. Despite your repeated promises to yourself, do you find yourself putting off starting your new habit?

2. Why do you do that, second?

3. Is it the difficulty you have starting a new habit?

4. Can you use the two-minute rule to your advantage when forming new habits?

OBJECTIVES YOU WANT TO REACH

1. Reduce the difficult-for-me-to-start habits to two minutes or less

2. Start structuring your daily tasks so that it takes progressively more time to be able to carry out negative habits (reversing the 2-minute rule)

YOUR ACTION PLAN

1. Examine how to use the two-minute rule to start a new habit.

2. Create challenges using the habit-shaping method.

AN ACTION PLAN

1. From your habits scorecard, choose a new habit you want to start or one you have been trying to.

2. Follow the 2-minute rule. Start modestly, always.

3. Apply the habit-forming strategy. Start by establishing goals that are doable for you to achieve. For instance, I'll walk for 10 minutes tomorrow, then 20 minutes the day after that, etc. To make a solid start to your new habit, it's critical to go through that first hurdle.

SUMMARY

Making excellent habits simple to follow is the subject of the third law of behavior change. Repetition is a powerful tool for automating a behavior. To facilitate habit formation, we can use friction-reducing techniques and environmental design. The two-minute rule is an excellent method for putting an end to procrastination and for starting and maintaining a new habit.

Make it difficult to persist with your poor habits is the reversal of the third law, which is to make things simple. An action gets less appealing as the friction to perform it rises.

COMMITMENT INSTRUMENTS

James advises you to develop a commitment tool that will make it more difficult for you to engage in the undesirable habit. Making a commitment is deciding now to limit your future behavior and bad habits in order to maintain harmony with your positive routines.

You are in control of developing a commitment tool to assist you in maintaining your positive routines and breaking bad ones. For instance, purchase snacks in single servings rather than in bulk to assist you reduce snacking. You can resist temptation with the use of commitment tools. Giving your coworker your phone for two hours while you concentrate on writing your report without interruptions is a fantastic example.

Make an effective commitment tool so that breaking it requires more effort or costs more money than taking the activity. You are more likely to keep your promise if, for example, you pay in advance for a workout class at the gym because you want to begin a new habit of becoming fit and healthy.

Making an undesirable habit difficult or unfeasible to perform is the greatest approach to break it. The decisions you make can help to determine whether a good habit lasts over time. James Clear conducted a survey of his readers to find out whether they had any quick, simple behaviors that helped them form better, more lasting habits. He obtained some intriguing outcomes. The list below includes a few of them. They might offer you some inspiration.

Nutrition: Eat less calories by using smaller dishes.

Get blackout curtains and turn off the television in your bedroom so you can sleep.

Be productive by using email filters to empty your inbox and turning off your phone.

Purchase a supportive chair or a standing desk for general health.

Setting up automated bill payment and cutting cable.

Using technology to help you is a smart approach to automate healthy habits and get rid of the bad ones. When it comes to habits that happen infrequently, such as automatically buying medicines or stopping social media browsing with a website blocker, technology is especially helpful. By automating some aspects of your life, you may focus your time and effort on activities that are more important to you.

The drawback of automation is that it makes things so simple that we establish undesirable habits because it's so convenient to do so. as when you binge-watch a television show on Netflix because it automatically starts playing the next episode. Using social media instead of going for a walk when you have a break is another example. It is up to us to use the advice and techniques that have been provided thus far to make walking as friction-free as possible because reaching for your phone is so much simpler.

Automation may make good habits inevitable and bad ones unavoidable when it works in your favor.

IMPORTANT TAKEAWAYS FROM THIS CHAPTER

1. The third law of behavior change is inverted, meaning that making something difficult will make it easier.

2. An action becomes less appealing when there is greater friction involved in performing it.

3. Design a commitment tool to make it more difficult to engage in your undesirable habit. You can get help from technology.

4. Reevaluate your decisions to make sure your positive habit sticks around.

DETERMINE RELATED PROBLEMS

1. Do you ever feel like you get into negative habits too quickly?

2. How can you stop yourself from developing unhealthy habits?

3. If you make a commitment to a good behavior and it costs you money to break it, are you more likely to stick with it?

OBJECTIVES YOU WANT TO REACH

1. Make it challenging to develop undesirable behaviors.

2. Maintain my positive routines.

YOUR ACTION PLAN

1. Create more resistance by adding more steps between me and my unhealthy habits.

2. Avoid letting technology cause me to develop negative habits.

3. Employ a commitment tool.

AN ACTION PLAN

1. What can you do to make it more difficult to engage in harmful habits? Give at least two examples.

2. Does the technology in your environment occasionally cause you to develop undesirable habits? How do you stop this? Give an instance.

3. Consider a commitment tool that would work for one of your habits and that you could implement.

Put it in writing.

PART FIVE:

THE 4TH LAW: MAKE IT SATISFYING

CH. 15: THE FUNDAMENTAL PRINCIPLE OF BEHAVIOR CHANGE

SUMMARY

The fourth law of behavior change proposed by James Clear, Make it Satisfying, is covered in this chapter as well as the two following it.

James tells the tale of public health worker Stephen Luby at the beginning of the chapter. In the late 1990s, Luby traveled to Karachi, Pakistan, with his team to address the public health crisis.

The widespread lack of handwashing habits among the populace is mostly to blame for the health issues in the neighborhood. They were able to properly wash their hands. Additionally, they were aware that washing their hands before to cooking was important, yet they either acted erratically or inconsistently when doing so.

Handwashing became more joyful when Luby and his staff, along with Proctor and Gamble, began to provide the neighborhood with what the inhabitants perceived as "premium" soap. Safeguard soap was popular among users, and as a result, handwashing habits grew more ingrained. Therefore, it began a new habit rather than just resulting in a shift in behavior.

The health of the local youngsters started to improve right away, and when researchers returned several years later, they discovered that locals had continued the practice.

This is only one illustration of how, as humans, we are more inclined to repeat an action if the experience is pleasurable. Even something as simple as washing one's hands with fragrant, foaming soap sends messages to the brain informing it that it is a pleasurable experience. Your brain is stimulated by this positive emotion to recall and repeat the action that caused it.

Similar to this, our brains do not enjoy events that do not fulfill us or provide us joyful feelings. It does not understand the necessity for wanting that action to be repeated as a

result. Simply said, we subconsciously repeat the things we enjoy doing and avoid doing the things we find unpleasant.

This takes us to the fourth law of behavior change, which is to make the habit loop satisfying.

REWARD TYPES: IMMEDIATE AND DELAYED

According to Clear, we tend to look for immediate satisfaction rather than merely any kind of fulfillment. The "immediate-return environment" that animals inhabit is one in which decisions have immediate effects. The "delayed-return environment" in which people live, however, is particularly prevalent in modern culture. This implies that we may not always perceive the immediate results of our activities in the here and now. For instance, if you exercise or eat a healthy meal today in an effort to reduce weight, you won't notice effects for a few weeks or perhaps months.

Our early ancestors were accustomed to receiving rapid gratification. The future was far off, and the biggest concern was how to survive in the here and now. As a result, we continue to favor immediate pleasure. This is bad news for forming habits!

Bad habits provide you rapid gratification, immediate rewards, and delayed repercussions. For instance, the detrimental effects of smoking or binge eating only become apparent over time.

Good behaviors typically have the opposite effect. The result is not satisfying or delightful right away. The satisfying result is the one we are striving for in the end.

Because the present moment takes precedence in our brains, instant gratification—good or bad—often prevails when decisions must be made. Understanding how our brains are programmed to seek for instant gratification may aid in our ability to learn to accept delayed gratification.

We will reap the rewards in the long term if we take advantage of human nature (the desire for instant satisfaction) by including a small amount of immediate pleasure into the process of habit building. Make it satisfying right away, in other words.

By rewarding yourself with small pleasures like a massage after a couple of gym sessions, you may make the new habit delightful. This enables you to stay motivated for a longer period of time until you start to notice results.

IMPORTANT TAKEAWAYS FROM THIS CHAPTER

1. Unhealthy behaviors provide us instant enjoyment since we can see outcomes.

2. The results of excellent practices only become apparent over time

3. Adding a small amount of instant pleasure to a healthy habit can have long-term benefits.

4. Small rewards such as reinforcements can keep you on track.

DETERMINE RELATED PROBLEMS

1. Do you tend to want immediate pleasure for the majority of your actions?

2. Do you believe that rewarding yourself in some small way after finishing your habit will keep you motivated?

3. Do you treat yourself after a good behavior is finished?

OBJECTIVES YOU WANT TO REACH

1. Even though the benefits may only be seen in the future, I want to make sure that my new habit is satisfying and delightful.

2. It will be in my best interest to come up with creative ideas for how I might use short-term rewards to motivate me toward my longer-term objectives.

YOUR ACTION PLAN

1. Look for methods to enjoy my habit.

2. You can also improve your thinking. You might get more satisfaction if you alter the way you see the same behaviors.

AN ACTION PLAN

1. Come up with a list of modest prizes that you may use to motivate yourself and give you short-term gratification while you work to establish new habits. Rewards might range from drinking wine or reading a new book by your favorite author to using the habit

stacking technique to incorporate a pleasant action after you have finished practicing your habit.

2. Use reinforcements like a habit tracker (see Chapter Sixteen) to make the reward satisfying. Seeing your successes is beneficial and a fantastic visual motivator. Observing your development helps you to maintain your identity as a fit or healthy person.

SUMMARY

It's one thing to start a good habit, but for many of us, maintaining it after a few weeks or even days is difficult. We like to see proof of our accomplishments as humans. James offers a few methods for helping us retain a visual record of our routines.

The "Paper Clip Strategy" is one such tactic. This is a straightforward method for tracking your development visually. Keep an empty jar next to the one with paperclips, marbles, or something similar to illustrate this tactic. You transfer an item from the full jar to the empty jar after each time you engage in your new behavior. This method of tracking your development visually is not only gratifying, but it also supports behavior reinforcement.

HABIT MONITOR

Using the "habit tracker" is another approach to gauge your progress. This monitors whether you engaged in a habit. An easy way to keep track of your new habits is to mark off the days on a calendar when you follow them. The Laws of Behavior Change are covered by habit monitoring, which is a particularly efficient technique because:

1. **It is clear** – By creating a series of visual cues, such as the Xs, on your calendar, it is clear that you should continue operating following your habit. The proof that you maintain your habits is constantly in front of you.

2. **It is appealing** – Habit tracking shows the results of your efforts, which inspires you to keep going. You are motivated to fill in the empty squares when you see the filled-in squares followed by the open squares.

3. **It is gratifying** – Checking things off our to-do lists makes many of us feel good. Similar to tracking your habits, adding those Xs makes you feel rewarded as you observe your improvement.

With habit tracking, you give the process more attention than the end result. Making a visual cue can be encouraging because you can see your improvement and the act of tracking your success itself makes you feel good.

ONLY SOME PEOPLE ARE FANS OF TRACKING.

Because it seems like more work and requires two habits, some people are reluctant to track. You are attempting to develop the first habit, and the second is to cultivate a tracking habit. Two things you should keep in mind.

However, Clear asserts that attempting to automate your tracking is an excellent method to make it simpler. Your habits may occasionally be monitored without your knowledge. For instance, your credit card account will show you how frequently you eat out, and your smartwatch can track your movements. You can evaluate automated data once a week or once a month.

Not every habit needs to be tracked manually. James advises restricting it to your most crucial habit in order to keep track of it regularly. Additionally, it's a good idea to record your behavior right away. When the habit is finished, that's your cue to record it.

James advises combining your habit tracking with the habit stacking strategy from Chapter 5. The equation would be as follows:

I will track my habit after I [do my present behavior].

WHAT TO DO IF A STREAK OF GOOD HABITS ENDS

Every habit streak eventually comes to an end. It's critical to have a recovery strategy in place in case you falter. Now and again, life will divert you from your course. You never know what catastrophe or emergency might prevent you from carrying out your habit on that day or at that moment in the future. Whatever transpires, James advises, the most crucial thing is to make sure you never make the same mistake twice.

This is crucial because, much too frequently, we are prone to repeating errors after making one. When you break a habit, get back into it as soon as possible to avoid losing it and establishing a new one from scratch.

Following an all-or-nothing cycle is unnecessary when forming and maintaining a new habit. If you make a mistake, carefully pick up your habit immediately. Or at least try to complete even a small portion of it; for instance, even if you don't feel like working out, it is still preferable not to show there. Being present is preferable to disrupting your cycle. Recall the 1% improvement compounding theory. At the very least, attendance retains your cumulative gains from earlier outcomes. Additionally, it confirms your identify as, say, a fit person.

MEASURING INCORRECTLY

Your habit streak may end if you are trying to figure out what to track or when to track it. Don't accept less than what you are measuring for. Always keep in mind your goals and the bigger picture.

Even though certain things cannot be quantified using statistics or figures, that does not imply that they are insignificant. Being purely motivated by a number, such as the weight you are attempting to drop on the scale, might be demoralizing. Additionally, take note of how your weight loss to date has also improved your skin and reduced the size of your waist by a few inches. Not just the weight on the scale, but also these are indications of your development.

Habit tracking can improve your habit behavior and give you proof that you are progressing in the right direction.

IMPORTANT TAKEAWAYS FROM THIS CHAPTER

1. Observing our development satisfies us and inspires us to maintain our routines.

2. We can use a habit tracker to track our new habits.

3. It's critical to maintain a habit streak. If you err once, try to pick up where you left off. Don't ever miss twice.

4. Measuring something does not necessarily imply that it is the sole way to monitor your development. Search for additional proof as well.

DETERMINE RELATED PROBLEMS

1. Are you the sort of person who enjoys monitoring their progress?

2. Do you track your development continuously? How do you gauge your effect?

3. Would habit monitoring serve as a motivator for you?

4. Has your habitual cycle ever been broken? What did you do in response? How did you reorient yourself?

5. Do you find tracking your success in forming new habits to be tedious?

6. Would keeping track of your behavior streak with a habit tracker be helpful? And how would you use automation to help you with some of the tracking?

OBJECTIVES YOU WANT TO REACH

1. I hope to maintain my new habit.

2. I want to learn how to keep tabs on my development.

YOUR ACTION PLAN

1. Decide which of your habits you want to monitor.

2. Choose the habit-tracking technique that will work best for you.

3. Gather the necessary resources, such as an appropriate app or calendar.

4. Create a statement for your habit stacking and tracking.

5. Make a mental note to look for further proof of your improvement in addition to the figures.

AN ACTION PLAN

1. Make daily updates to your habit tracker.

2. Introspection: What are your thoughts about this? Does monitoring require more effort, energy, or time on your part, or does it make it easier for you to maintain your new habit?

CH. 17: HOW A PARTNER IN ACCOUNTABILITY CAN TRANSFORM EVERYTHING

SUMMARY

Making a habit satisfying is the fourth law of behavior modification, and the converse is making a habit unsatisfactory. We swiftly learn not to repeat mistakes when we are forced to take responsibility for them. Add an immediate penalty to break poor habits, and watch how unattractive it becomes.

Punishment can occasionally alter a person's behavior, particularly a harmful habit. For instance, if you have a bad practice of paying your bills after they are due, you will eventually incur a large sum of money in late fees. You start paying your bills on time to avoid having to make this extra amount each time you pay a bill late.

Your behavior can alter if you raise the price of your poor habit relative to the price of your action. Making a "habit contract" is one technique to give a poor habit an immediate consequence.

HABIT AGREEMENT

People are held accountable by laws and contracts, and society follows certain laws that are essential to maintaining order. The same manner, by making a habit contract, we may keep ourselves accountable. You should put your commitment to your new behavior in writing along with the consequences of breaking it.

The next stage is to find a partner who will sign the contract with you and function as your accountability partner.

Even if you don't have a formal agreement in writing, having an accountability partner can still be beneficial. The accountability partner can be a buddy, your spouse, your trainer, someone you exercise with, or simply someone who follows you around or keeps an eye on you.

It can be really motivating to be aware of onlookers. It is only human nature for us to be concerned with what other people think.

IMPORTANT TAKEAWAYS FROM THIS CHAPTER

1. We are less likely to repeat harmful habits if we make them painful or unsatisfying.

2. Having a companion who holds us accountable makes it easier to incur an immediate cost when we break our excellent routines.

3. An effective inducement to guarantee that we maintain our habits is a habit contract.

DETERMINE RELATED PROBLEMS

1. Do you believe that a habit contract would be an excellent tool for holding yourself accountable?

2. Would having a partner in accountability be beneficial to you?

OBJECTIVES YOU WANT TO REACH

1. I want to set up a procedure to hold myself responsible for my habits.

YOUR ACTION PLAN

1. List the people you believe would make good accountability partners for you.

2. Choose one or two people and inquire as to their interest in serving as your accountability partners.

3. Establish a habit contract with appropriate consequences for breaking it.

AN ACTION PLAN

1. Create your habit contract and have it approved. Your habit contract should include a list of your target, goal, the repercussions of failing to achieve those goals, and your accountability (penalty).

2. Consideration: Is your habit contract effective for you? Make sure to review your habit contracts to determine whether they are keeping you to your good habits, preventing you from your good habits, and preventing you from your bad habits as intended.

PART SIX:

ADVANCED TACTICS HOW TO GO FROM BEING MERELY GOOD TO BEING TRULY GREAT

CH 18: THE TRUTH ABOUT TALENT (WHEN GENES MATTER AND WHEN THEY DON'T)

SUMMARY

The fourth law, "make it unsatisfying," which is the opposite of the fifth law, was completed in the previous chapter. James offers readers a few strategies in the book's concluding section to help them advance from being good to outstanding.

When you decide to change a habit, the habits you pick are simpler to keep up if they complement your inherent skills and interests. Our genes heavily influence how we act and what we do, even though we are all born with unique traits and abilities.

Sometimes, the alignment of our genes with our behaviour works in our favor. For instance, having the gene for height can help you if you want to be a professional basketball player. But being tall might not be an asset if you want to become a professional gymnast. Have you ever seen a gymnast that is seven feet tall?

While your genes may give you the chance to develop the ability of your choice, this potential is only valid if what you want to achieve aligns with that advantage. When they do coincide, habit formation may be most advantageous. But keep in mind that your surroundings or context may have an impact on this.

According to James, you must be aware of your personality in order to increase your chances of success and make your habit more gratifying.

YOUR CHARACTER AND YOUR ROUTINE

Your DNA greatly influences your behavior. They also contribute to your propensity towards a particular personality. Five personality characteristics have a hereditary basis. The five categories of qualities, such as extroversion, conscientiousness, and so on, are covered in the exercises below. Search the list for the behaviors you are aware of in

yourself. These actions have an impact on the habits you develop and the level of satisfaction you derive from them.

For instance, agreeableness is one of the five qualities. People that are genetically prone to this attribute are typically courteous and friendly, and they cherish social connections. These are the ones who will naturally write thank-you cards as a habit. As a result, some people may find it simpler to maintain certain routines due to our deeply ingrained behaviors. It is preferable to develop habits that suit your personality. Instead of doing what everyone else is doing, decide to develop the habits that work best for you.

You can make your habits more pleasurable by modifying them to fit your personality. Additionally, you are more likely to appreciate doing what comes effortlessly. For instance, if you are talented in a particular area, you will perform better and win praise from others. You get more driven to improve because of this. You advance more quickly the more awards you receive.

Selecting the proper habit makes growth simpler. However, how can you choose the best habit? According to Clear, this can be accomplished through making mistakes. You should first investigate (study various concepts and options) to improve this. Utilize it if you locate anything that will work for you and you are successful at it. The "explore/exploit tradeoff" refers to this.

As you consider your alternatives, The following questions will help you better understand the behaviors that satisfy you.

• Do I believe that this hobby is more enjoyable than work? Do I find this enjoyable while others criticize it?

• Do I tend to lose track of time when I'm doing this activity? Does it cause me to experience flow? (Flow is the mental state that occurs when a person is entirely concentrated on what they are doing and loses track of anything else. It is the location of your peak performance).

• In what field or activity do I excel over others regarding results?

• What comes naturally to me, and what do I feel natural doing? What gives me joy and makes me feel most like myself?

Some persons are fortunate enough to be presented with favorable opportunities. Some folks have that kind of luck. Create your luck if you don't think you have it. Everybody excels in something. Concentrate on it and master it to the point where you stand out. Create a game that is appropriate for you, in other words. Focus on one area of expertise until you are the greatest at it.

Our genes help us identify our areas of strength and the things we should focus on and steer clear of. Consequently, it is vital to comprehend your nature. Understanding your personality will help you decide on the best course of action. It is better for you long term and more gratifying to choose behaviors that fit with your inherent abilities and personality.

IMPORTANT TAKEAWAYS FROM THIS CHAPTER

1. Decide where you would be able to compete best in order to increase your chances of success.

2. Choosing the appropriate habit makes growth more manageable.

3. If you use your genes to your advantage, they can be pretty helpful. They can help you identify the things you should work hard on, but they don't always make working hard unnecessary.

4. Pick a habit that plays to your strengths and is therefore simpler to maintain.

DETERMINE RELATED PROBLEMS

1. Do you identify with the statement, "Sometimes I try to form habits that go against my personality"?

2. Do you find it harder to maintain these practices than I do?

OBJECTIVES YOU WANT TO REACH

1. I must align my habits with my personality or natural abilities.

2. Do you find it harder to maintain these practices than I do?

GOALS YOU'D LIKE TO ACCOMPLISH

1. I must adjust my habits to reflect my personality or my inherent abilities.

2. When I perceive behaviors that are inconsistent with my personality, I try to alter the habit to fit who I am.

YOUR ACTION PLAN

1. Match behavior Starting with my personality, please.

2. Establish routines that suit my personality

3. Employ the explore/exploit technique to determine my best options.

AN ACTION PLAN

1. Locate a personality test online (several to choose from) and finish the one you want.

2. See the list below and mark the characteristics that best describe your conduct. Each element is characterized on a scale, with the left side representing the description that best fits the characteristic and the right side representing the opposite.

a. Being receptive to new things, ranging from being inquisitive and creative to being cautious and reliable.

b. Conscientiousness ranges from efficient and orderly to laid-back and impulsive.

c. Extroversion: from sociable and extroverted to lonely and reserved (extroverts vs. introverts, as you probably already know).

d. Being agreeable ranges from being kind and sympathetic to being stern and distant.

e. Neuroticism: ranges from confident, serene, and stable to worried and sensitive.

3. Select the opportunities and behaviors that are best for you after getting a deeper understanding of your personality and behavioral qualities.

CHAPTER 19: THE GOLDILOCKS RULE; HOW TO MAINTAIN MOTIVATION AT WORK AND IN LIFE

SUMMARY

As you have probably already discovered, maintaining your habits over the long term can be challenging. Why do some people find it easier than others to maintain their routines?

Their capacity to maintain motivation is the key. Only challenges that fall inside an "optimal zone of difficulty" are appealing to our brains. According to research, we will stay motivated if we work on challenges we can handle.

Conversely, if something is too difficult, you may lose drive. If something is too simple, you may get bored. The "Goldilocks Rule" should be followed if you want to be happy. This principle states that when people work on difficult activities just outside their existing capabilities, they are most motivated. fairly simple. not too simple. Exactly right.

Just enough successes and blunders will keep you striving and inspired, respectively. Keep your new habit as simple as possible to ensure that you stick with it. Once the habit has been formed, you can adjust or add new tasks to keep yourself interested and motivated.

FOCUSING ONESELF

Boring can come from repeating the same actions. Everyone experiences periods of low motivation, but those who persevere and achieve their goals are the ones who can maintain their motivation despite boredom.

Solid performance demands a lot of effort and practicing might get monotonous. The same old routine gets boring after a while. According to Clears, boredom—not failure—is one of the biggest dangers to success. The elements of surprise are constantly rewarding when you encounter something new. This is referred to as a changeable reward by psychologists.

Everybody has days when they want to give up a new habit or anything else they start. But if we can overcome those obstacles, we shall triumph. According to James, that sets professionals apart from amateurs; professionals "keep to the schedule, while amateurs "let life get in the way."

Ultimately, if a habit is genuinely essential to you, you will stick with it regardless of your challenges or feelings. You "have to fall in love with boredom" to become outstanding at something.

IMPORTANT TAKEAWAYS FROM THIS CHAPTER

1. Working on problems that are manageable in difficulty helps you stay motivated.

2. The Goldilocks Principle—not too easy, not too hard, but just right—is the finest place to be.

3. One of the most significant obstacles to our achievement may be boredom brought on by repetition. The key is to maintain motivation.

4. You must find ways to push past boredom to become outstanding at something.

DETERMINE RELATED PROBLEMS

1. Do you occasionally become bored while forming a new habit?

2. How do you break the monotony?

3. Do you stop engaging in your habit when you get bored? Do you instead motivate yourself with minor obstacles or rewards?

OBJECTIVES YOU WANT TO REACH

1. I wish to overcome boredom and maintain my motivation.

YOUR ACTION PLAN

1. Be on the lookout for new habits to develop.

2. Look for ways to maintain my motivation so I can go over the stage of boredom.

3. Modify/change my daily schedule to keep it fresh.

4. Add something new to my habitual pattern to break up the monotony.

AN ACTION PLAN

1. I've discovered effective strategies for overcoming boredom in my habitual pattern.

2. Describe your actions and their results.

CH 20: THE DOWNSIDE OF CREATING GOOD HABITS

SUMMARY

You must achieve a degree of proficiency at anything where you can carry out the steps so effortlessly that you don't even have to think about it. This is assisted by habits.

However, just like everything else, habits have advantages and disadvantages. The drawback of developing a habit is that we become so accustomed to performing the activity automatically that we may overlook small mistakes. Even if you practice the habit more frequently, you may not necessarily get better as you gain experience.

You cannot just blindly repeat actions in order to become an expert at something. For instance, when brushing your teeth, this might work. You can't really do much better there. You must mix instinctive habits with purposeful practice if you want to excel at something.

You must start forming the next habit as soon as you get the previous one under control. The habit (or skill) you have mastered is typically the starting point for moving on to the next phase of developing your skill set. One improvement is gradually built on top of another. Up until you achieve a higher level of performance, each habit builds on the one before it.

You must practice being aware of how you perform in order to continue to develop and sharpen your expertise over time. You can prevent falling into the trap of complacency by setting up a mechanism for reflection and revision.

Reviewing your progress and your present behaviors helps you make long-term improvements to your habits. You can identify any errors you are making or justifications for your lack of development through reflection and review. It enables you to assess whether or not your performance has improved.

James Clear explains how he personally employs two techniques for reflection and revision, both of which are effective for him. These consist of an annual assessment in which he considers the prior year and an integrity report following six months. In order to determine whether he is still on track to becoming the person he wants to be, he utilizes his integrity report to review his key principles and reflect on his identity.

These two reports aid James in avoiding falling back into previous routines when he is not paying attention. They assist him in determining whether he is on track or whether he needs to improve his routines and, if necessary, take on new challenges.

Reexamining one's identity is crucial in order to examine any outdated assumptions you still hold onto that are restricting your progress. Sometimes our attachment to one identity is so strong that when change is required, we struggle to adjust. Don't limit how you define yourself for the rest of your life. If the concept of who you believe yourself to be has changed, as it frequently does for people after retirement, you are lost. Now who are you?

Keep in mind that your role and your identity are distinct concepts as you try to cope with these identity losses. Your identity does not alter if your role—for example, that of a company's CEO—does. You continue to be the kind of person who constructs and produces things. Your identity is malleable and subject to change as conditions do.

IMPORTANT TAKEAWAYS FROM THIS CHAPTER

1. Habits aid in the acquisition of new skills, but we must watch out lest they become so automatic that we lose sight of our areas for improvement.

2. Regularly thinking back and analyzing our development helps us stay aware of where we are and where we can grow.

3. Watch out for becoming too attached to one identity and becoming unable to adapt as and when necessary.

DETERMINE RELATED PROBLEMS

1. What drawback did you experience once you mastered a habit or skill?

2. Do you have a system in place for reviewing and reflecting?

3. Could you change who you are to fit shifting circumstances?

GOALS YOU WANT TO ACHIEVE

1.1 want to make sure I don't become comfortable.

2. I also want to put out all of my effort to be the best version of myself and avoid getting entangled in self-identities that no longer accurately represent me.

YOUR ACTION PLAN

1. I'll start using a reflect and review technique to prevent complacency.

2. Assess the habits I have developed.

3. Evaluate whether they have assisted me in staying loyal to who I am.

AN ACTION PLAN

1. Think back on the previous year and respond to the following questions:

a. What was successful for you? What went wrong for you? What did you discover?

b. What fundamental principles guide your life? What fundamental principles guide your work? How are you currently acting morally? How can you improve your own standards going forward?

2. Decide whether to reflect and review once a month or once a year.

CONCLUSION:

THE SECRET TO RESULTS THAT LAST

This workbook offers you a variety of tactics to help you form and keep good habits while getting rid of undesirable ones.

Our behaviors have a significant impact on how our lives and identities are shaped. Many of our daily actions are within their control. Our success will come from knowing how to create positive habits and get rid of negative ones.

The book Atomic Habits demonstrates how even small changes may have a significant impact on our lives and help us achieve our objectives. A small improvement of 1 percent adds enough to make a huge effect.

We are better able to keep these excellent habits and accomplish our goals when we concentrate on creating good systems to create positive habits. We make tiny but consistent enhancements to our systems to make them more effective.

Four Rules for Behavior Change is a straightforward set of guidelines we may use to create healthy habits. Make a habit evident to make it easier to perform, and make it appealing to encourage you to begin. Find ways to make a new habit easier to start, and if you find it difficult to maintain, attempt to make it more pleasant to keep yourself motivated.

Use the opposite of the Four Laws to make the bad habit invisible, unappealing, tough, and unsatisfying if you're trying to break one.

Developing new habits is a constant process. You may create healthier habits, keep them up, and accomplish your goals if you work consistently and with dedication.

We hope that while working through this workbook, you got the chance to put some of the suggestions into practice in your own life.

We wish you well as you establish new habits. And if you haven't already, do it right away!

writing letters to him. Now when she looked back, she knew she shouldn't have been so patient.

Wilson supported abiogenesis primarily because Wilson believed Calvin and Elizabeth were dating, and Avery also liked the difficult situation it put Donatti in. Avery learned that Calvin and Elizabeth were dating via the gossip at Hastings.

Wilson had intended to meet Elizabeth in person and was aware that she was a woman until Calvin unexpectedly passed away. Due to inaccurate publications about Calvin's death and their connection, Avery assumed Elizabeth wasn't close to him.

Elizabeth had left the funeral so swiftly that Avery, who was present, was unable to meet her. Elizabeth yelled out that she did completely and never ceased loving him, contrary to what she had imagined. They clutched each other while crying in sorrow.

W

ATOMIC

HABITS

An Easy & Proven Way

To Build Good Habits &

Break Bad Ones

JAMES CLEAR

Tiny Changes,

Remarkable

Result

An Implementation Guide and Workbook

Based on James Clear's Book